WEIGHT LOSS AND MANAGEMENT

Your Comprehensive Handbook for Sustainable Health and Well-Being

ALIU BABATUNDE

Weight Loss and Management

ISBN: 9798867768119

DEDICATION

To my parents,

Their constant devotion, love, and support for my wellbeing have served as the cornerstone of my path. This work has been motivated by your support and conviction in my abilities. This book is proof of the knowledge you have given me regarding health, resiliency, and the value of living a well-rounded life. I am grateful that you are my guiding lights.

CONTENTS

ACKNOWLEDGMENTS

I would want to express my profound gratitude to everyone who helped make "Weight Loss and Management" a reality. Your encouragement, commitment, and support have been invaluable in the development of this guide. I am grateful that you have trusted me to be your guide on the road to a better and happier life, readers who are embarking on this adventure. I hope this eBook empowers you on your wellness path and encourages good transformations.

INTRODUCTION

The importance of weight control cannot be emphasized in a society where people value their health and well-being above all else. It is the foundation of a happier, healthier existence and the guide pointing us in the direction of a vibrant, self-assured future. Introducing "Weight Loss and Management," a vital manual that helps you understand the complex web of weight and provides you with the information, resources, and tactics you need to change the way you interact with your body.

The Significance of Weight Management

A fundamental concept is at the core of this eBook: managing weight involves more than just looking at numbers on a scale or trying to achieve an idealized body type. It's about protecting your general wellbeing, preserving your health, and tending to the structure that contains your inner being. Your decisions about weight affect not just your physical well-being but also your emotional and mental stability. You are starting on a path to being a healthier, happier version of yourself by realizing how important weight control is. here. Finding the Goal of This eBook "Weight Loss and Management" has two goals in mind. Its primary goal is to clarify the science behind weight management and provide you with the knowledge you need to make wise decisions regarding your health. You will learn more about the specifics of exercise, diet, and metabolism and how these aspects interact with one another to help you achieve your weight loss goals. Second, this eBook offers you real-world tactics, advice, and support, acting as an understanding and helpful guide. It is intended to support you in creating a sustainable strategy, setting realistic objectives, and navigating the frequently difficult route to weight reduction and management. You will learn about the "what," "why," and "how" of reaching and maintaining a healthy weight in these pages.

What's Awaiting You

The following chapters contain plenty of evidence-based knowledge and practical guidance. You will learn about the science of balanced nutrition, create specific fitness plans, and understand the importance of having a positive outlook. We will also clarify myths surrounding weight loss, acknowledge your accomplishments, and arm you with the skills you require to overcome challenges. Together, we'll set out on a journey to a greater, more satisfying life—not just a healthy weight. After finishing this book, you will have the skills and self-assurance necessary to start, continue, and enjoy your own personal transformation. This eBook is intended only to provide guidance; the journey is up to you to take.

Understanding the Effects of Weight

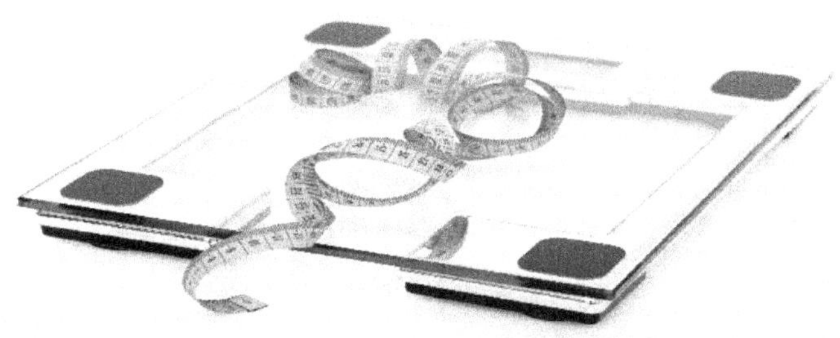

Gaining knowledge about the meaning and concept of weight is essential if we are to make progress toward better health and wellbeing. Weight is a reflection of our lifestyle, our decisions, and our general health rather than merely a number on a scale. Our starting point is covered in this chapter, where we explore the complexities of weight, how it's calculated, the effects of being overweight or obese, and the myths surrounding weight and body image.

i. Defining Weight and How It's Calculated

In its most basic form, weight is the measurement of the gravitational force applied to an object, in this example, your body. Usually, weight is expressed in quantities like pounds or kilograms. Although stepping onto a scale gives you a numerical description of your body's gravitational force, it is not a complete picture.

In order to comprehend the meaning of your weight, you must first realize that your body is made up of several substances, such as water, bone, fat, and muscle. A more complete picture of your health takes into account not just your total weight but also how these components are distributed. Your well-being, physical fitness, and overall health can all be significantly impacted by your body composition.

ii. Talking About the Health Consequences of Being Obese or Overweight

Almost every system in your body can be negatively impacted by being overweight or obese, which can have a significant impact on your health. Being overweight increases the strain on your bones, joints, and organs. It also raises your chance of a number of illnesses, such as the following:

• **Cardiovascular disease:** Being overweight boosts the risk of stroke, high blood pressure, and heart disease.

• **Diabetes:** One of the main risk factors for the onset of diabetes and insulin resistance is obesity.

• Respiratory problems: Obesity can cause disorders such as diminished lung function and sleep apnea.

• **Joint issues:** Carrying more weight can strain your joints more, which can result in diseases like osteoarthritis.

• **Mental health issues:** Higher rates of anxiety and depression are linked to overweight and obesity.

The important role of weight control as a means of achieving improved health and wellbeing is highlighted by the knowledge of the health risks associated with being overweight.

iii. Clearing Up Frequently Held Myths Regarding Weight and Body Image

There are a lot of myths and misconceptions about weight, body image, and health. Clearing up these misconceptions is crucial to promoting a positive relationship with our bodies. Here are a few widespread misunderstandings:

• **The myth:** "A lower number on the scale means better health." Truth: Being healthy involves much more than just weight. A vital influence is played by body composition, nutrition, physical activity, and other factors.

• **The myth that "all fat is bad." Truth:** Not all fats are created equal. For the proper operation of your body and general wellbeing, you need healthy fats.

• **Myth:** "Dieting is the only way to lose weight." Reality: Leading a balanced and healthful lifestyle is the key to sustainable weight management instead of dieting.

By clearing these myths, we can encourage a more compassionate and realistic perception of our bodies, opening the door to a more health-conscious method of managing weight.

We will look into the science behind weight, go further into the variables that affect it, and gain knowledge to help us make wise decisions regarding our health in the trip ahead. Although it's not always simple, the path to weight loss and management is one that's worthwhile taking. Now that we have more information and a better understanding of weight and its effects, let's proceed.

The science of weight loss

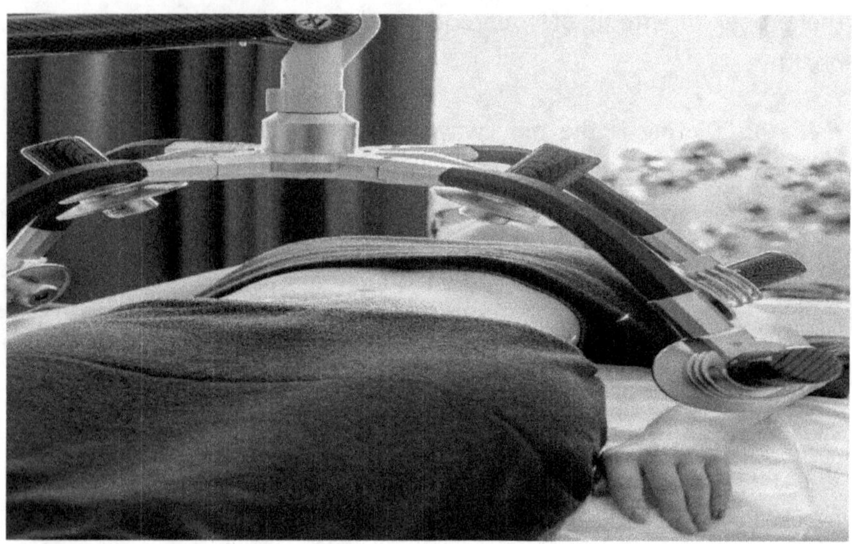

It's crucial that one understands the science of weight loss and management before beginning any successful journey. This chapter explores the basic concepts of energy balance, metabolism, and calories in order to shed light on weight loss strategies. We'll also look at the reasons behind the body's fat storage and burning processes as well as the influence of heredity on how each of us manages our weight.

ii. Explaining the Basics of Calories, Metabolism, and Energy Balance

The principles of energy balance, metabolism, and calories are fundamental to managing weight. Let's breakdown:

• **Energy:** Energy in the form of calories is obtained from the food and drinks we eat and drink. Maintenance calories are the number of calories your body requires to stay at its present weight. Weight growth occurs when you consume more calories than your body needs, and weight loss occurs when you consume fewer calories than your body needs.

• **Metabolism:** Your metabolism is the collection of chemical reactions that take place in your body in order to sustain life. It consists of two primary parts: basal metabolic rate (BMR) and physical activity. BMR is the amount of calories your body requires in order to sustain basic bodily functions like breathing and digestion, while physical activity is the amount of calories burned during physical activity and exercise.

iii. Genetics' Part in Managing Weight

Genetics influence how your body is predisposed to various aspects of managing your weight, such as:

• **Appetite:** A person's tendency to eat a certain amount and type of food depends on how their genes regulate their hunger and appetite.

• **Fat Storage:** Genetics can affect where fat is stored in the body; some people are more likely than others to store fat in particular places.

Genetics can influence events, but it cannot decide your fate. Genetic variables can be positively influenced, if not completely overruled, by a healthy lifestyle that includes exercise and proper diet.

Knowing the science of weight loss gives you the power to make wise decisions regarding your diet, exercise regimen, and way of life. It's an essential phase in your quest to reach and keep a healthy weight.

Realistic Goal-Setting

Setting attainable objectives is the first step towards effective weight loss and management. This chapter will cover the essential parts of goal-setting, such as the significance of setting realistic and long-term objectives, useful advice for creating and monitoring your goals, and psychological factors that affect the duration of your journey.

i. Determining the Significance of Creating Realistic and Long-Term Weight Loss Objectives

Establishing objectives is an essential first step in managing your weight. Setting attainable and long-term goals is just as important, though. This is the reason why:

• **Achievability:** Unattainable objectives, such as severe weight loss that happens quickly, can be demoralizing and unsustainable. Establishing attainable goals keeps your motivation high and improves your chances of success.

• Sustainability: The ultimate aim is long-term prosperity. Sustainable weight loss entails making long-term lifestyle adjustments and making improvements gradually and steadily.

Setting long-term, attainable goals helps you avoid regaining weight by positioning yourself for long-term success.

ii. Advice on Creating Goals and Monitoring Your Progress

Careful preparation and monitoring are necessary when setting goals that work. Take into account the following advice to improve your goal-setting procedure:

• **Be Particular:** Clearly state your objectives. Rather to just stating, "I want to lose weight," be more specific about how much weight you want to drop and when.

• **Measurable:** Put numbers on your list of objectives. Track your progress with data or numbers. For instance, set a weekly goal of losing 1-2 pounds.

• **Realistic**: Make sure your objectives are difficult but doable. Take into account your tastes, way of life, and any potential roadblocks.

• **Time-Bound:** Give your objectives a deadline. This makes you feel more pressed for time and keeps you on course.

• **Make both short- and long-term objectives:** Divide your journey to weight control into smaller, more achievable objectives. Realizing these.

iii. The Goal-Setting Process' Psychological Aspect

Setting goals is a psychological activity in addition to a mathematical one. The following psychological factors may impact your achievement:

• **Mentality:** Foster a growth mentality by having faith in your capacity to adapt and advance. Recognize that obstacles are a part of the path and treat yourself with kindness.

• **Motivation:** Recognize the internal and external forces driving you. Motivated by one's own values and aspirations, internal drive originates from inside. External drive is the result of outside influences such as praises or awards.

• **Mental Resilience:** View failures as chances to improve and learn. One of the most important components of long-term success is the capacity to overcome setbacks.

You may improve your capacity to persevere, maintain motivation, and navigate the ups and downs of your weight control journey by taking the psychological aspects of goal planning into account.

Remember that your goals are the guiding stars that will enlighten your path as you embark on this new chapter of your trip. You are giving yourself the best chance of long-term success in weight loss and control by creating objectives that are both practical and sustainable as well as comprehending the psychological aspects of goal creation.

Nutrition for Weight Loss

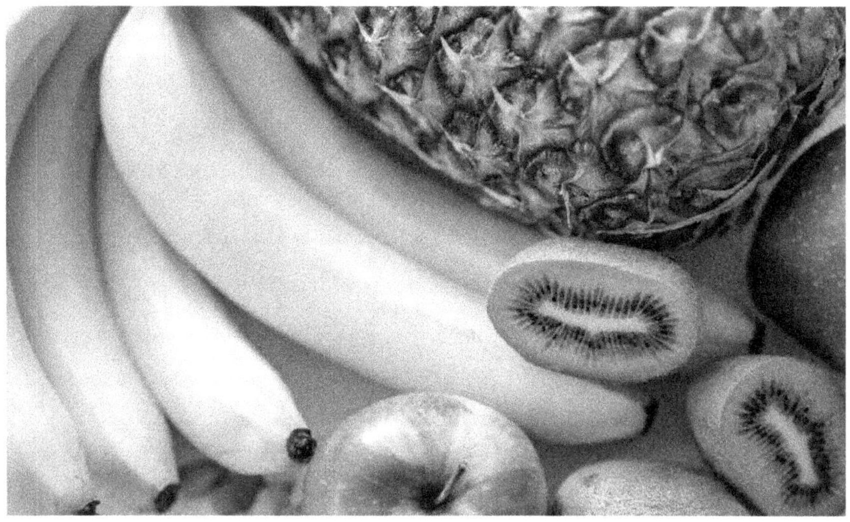

A healthy, well-balanced diet is the basis of effective weight management. The importance of a healthy, balanced diet, the function of macronutrients (carbohydrates, proteins, and fats), and an examination of micronutrients (vitamins and minerals) are just a few of the topics we'll cover in this chapter on nutrition for weight loss. We'll also go over portion control and efficient meal planning techniques to help you on your weight management pursuit.

i. The Value of a Healthful, Balanced Diet

A healthy, well-balanced diet is essential for effective weight management. This is why it's so important:

• **Density of nutrients**: Essential nutrients are provided by a balanced diet, which also reduces extra energy. Foods high in nutrients provide the greatest amount of vitamins, minerals, and other vital elements per energy, hence enhancing general well-being.

• **The satisfaction:** Eating a diverse range of meals from a balanced diet can make you feel content and full. This may lessen the desire to go overboard.

• **Sustainable development:** Long-term maintenance of a balanced diet is possible. Extreme limitations or crash diets are frequently problematic and result in weight gain.

ii. Going over macronutrients (proteins, fats, and carbohydrates) and micronutrients (minerals and vitamins)

To make wise food choices decisions, one must comprehend the functions of macronutrients and micronutrients:

• **carbohydrates:** The main energy source for the body is carbohydrate. To maintain energy levels and prevent blood sugar spikes, choose healthier carbohydrates (whole grains, fruits, and vegetables) over simple sweets.

• **Proteins:** Tissue development and maintenance depend on proteins. They also add to the sensation of richness. Fish, poultry, lean meat cuts, beans, and dairy products are examples of lean protein sources.

• **Fats:** Not all fats are created equal, yet fats are required for a number of body processes. Limit saturated and trans fats and concentrate on the good fats that can be found in the fruit, nuts, seeds, and olive oil.

• **Micronutrients:** Minerals and vitamins are essential for good bodily function and general health. They boost your energy levels and immune system, among other things. A diet rich in variety and balance supplies many of these vital micronutrients.

iii. Meal Preparation and Portion Control to Manage Weight

In your quest to manage your weight, efficient meal planning and portion control can make all the difference:

• **Meal Planning:** To make sure your meals and snacks fit your nutritional objectives, plan them in advance. Select complete, nutrient-dense foods that are high in important nutrients.

• **Portion Control:** Pay attention to how much is served. Eat off of smaller dishes, monitor your :Make an effort to eat meals that are rich in veggies, complex carbs, nutritious protein portions, and stay away from eating straight out of big containers. Overeating can be avoided by eating with awareness.

• **Balanced Meals, and healthy fats.** This level of balance can encourage steady blood sugar levels and satisfaction.

• **Hydration:** It's important to remember to stay hydrated. Water can help regulate hunger and is necessary for good health in general.

You are giving yourself the tools necessary to support your weight loss and management journey by emphasizing balanced and healthful diet, comprehending the function of macronutrients and micronutrients, and putting into practice efficient meal planning and portion control tactics.

We will build on the basis of good nutrition in the upcoming chapters as we investigate the science and techniques of successful weight management. Keep in mind that eating a good, balanced diet will give you greater health, vitality, and the ability to accomplish your goals rather than merely limiting what you can give up.

Physical Activity and Exercise

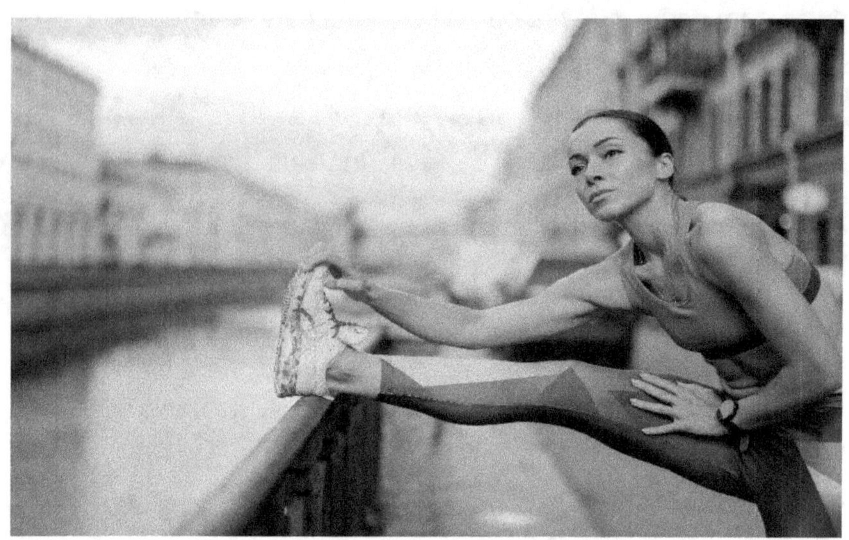

Engaging in physical activity is essential for effective weight management and is also a major way to improve general health. This chapter will cover the importance of physical activity for weight reduction, how to design a personalized exercise program for each person's tastes and lifestyle, and the advantages of combining cardiovascular, strength, and flexibility training for the best possible outcomes.

i. The Benefits of Exercise for Losing Weight and Improving General Health

Exercise is more than simply a way to burn calories; it's crucial for both weight loss and general health. Why it matters is as follows:

• **Calorie Expenditure:** Physical activity causes your body to burn more calories, which helps you lose weight by creating a calorie deficit.

• **Maintenance of Muscle:** Strong muscle mass is crucial for a healthy body composition and metabolism, and it may be preserved with regular exercise.

• **Control of Appetite:** Exercise helps control hunger hormones, which may lessen the need to overindulge.

• **Metabolic Health:** Exercise improves digestion, fatty acids levels, and blood sugar regulation.

• Mood and Well-Being: Exercise reduces stress and raises mood by releasing hormones known as end

ii. Formulating a Workout Program That Fits Personal Preferences and Lifestyles

The secret to effective exercise is to choose a method that fits your tastes and lifestyles. Here are some things to think about:

• **Type of Exercise:** Whether it's cycling, swimming, dancing, walking, jogging, or sports, pick things you enjoy doing. Consistency is more likely when it is enjoyable.

• **Frequency:** Try to work out on a daily basis. Although it is ideal to exercise most days of the week, even three or five times a week might be beneficial.

• **Duration:** Increase the length of your workouts gradually. As you gain endurance, increase from a manageable starting point and move forward.

• **Intensity:** Change up how hard you work out. Combine high- and moderate-intensity exercises to push your body and add variety to your routines.

• **Variety:** Avoid clear of boring workouts. To keep people interested and work different muscle areas, use a variety of exercises.

• **Adaptability:** The demands of life should not be met by your workout routine. Adjust your workouts to your energy levels and timetable.

iii. Integrating Flexibility, Strength, and Cardiovascular Training to Get the Best Outcomes

To get a comprehensive approach to physical activity, consider mixing several forms of exercise such as the following:

• **Aerobic or Cardiovascular Exercise:** This includes breathing and heart rate-raising exercises like cycling, swimming, and running. Enhancing cardiovascular health and burning calories are two benefits of cardiovascular exercise.

• **Resistance Training:** Increasing muscle mass with resistance training raises your resting metabolic rate in addition to increasing muscle mass. It is essential for preserving or increasing lean body mass.

• **Flexibility and Stretching:** Including stretching exercises increase general mobility, lowers the chance of injury, and improves flexibility.

Cardiovascular, strength, and flexibility training can help you improve your weight control efforts while providing a host of other health and fitness advantages for you to reap.

We will delve deeper into the realm of physical activity and exercise in the upcoming chapters, providing advice on how to create training plans, maintain motivation, and get beyond typical obstacles. Recall that physical activity is a necessary component of a better, more fulfilling life, not just a means to an end.

Myths and Facts About Weight Loss

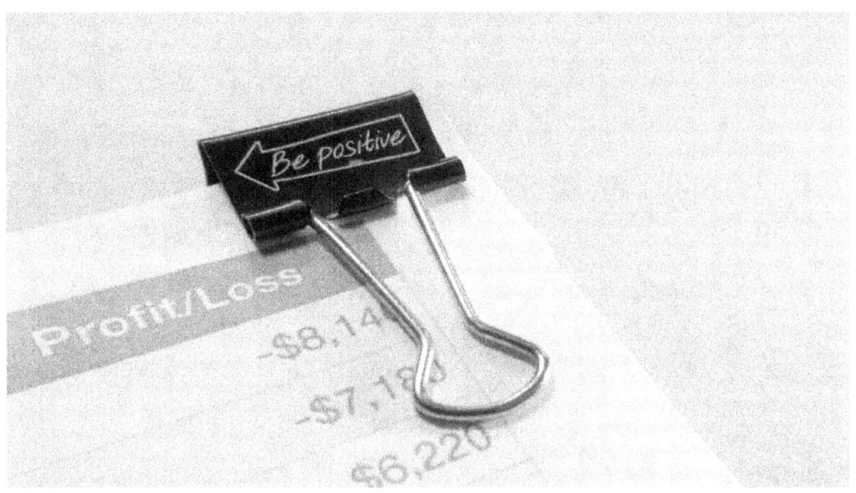

It can be difficult to tell truth from fiction in the wide realm of weight loss advice. Over the years, numerous misconceptions and fad diets have spread, offering simple, quick fixes for problems related to weight. This chapter will explain popular weight reduction myths and fad diets, offer evidence-based guidance on what actually works, and stress the significance of a sustainable and balanced approach to weight control.

Dispelling Flourishing Diet Myths and Common Weight Loss Myths

i. Myth: People Can Lose Weight Permanently with Crash Diets Fact: Although crash diets might cause rapid weight loss at first, they are not long-lasting and frequently cause a slowed metabolism, dietary shortages, and muscle loss. Usually, if regular eating patterns are restored, the lost weight is gained back.

ii. Myth: You Should Stay Clear of carbohydrates, The truth is that the body needs carbohydrates as a primary energy source. Aim for complex, high-fiber carbohydrates such as fruits, vegetables, and whole grains instead of removing them. They support general health and offer continuous energy.

iii. Myth: In order to lose weight, you must exercise excessively Truth: You don't have to spend hours every day at the gym to lose weight; exercise is beneficial for overall health. The more important factor in weight loss is what you eat. The goal is to eat a balanced diet, and exercise should support it.

Providing Information Based on Evidence on What Actually Works

i. Caloric Deficit: The Essential Idea The main factor in weight loss is a calorie deficit. You must consume fewer calories than you exert in order to lose weight. To enable steady, long-term weight loss, a persistent calorie deficit must be established.

Ii.Nutrition in Balance: Quality Counts Prioritize eating a diet rich in different kinds of nutrients and well-balanced. Make lean proteins, complex carbs, healthy fats, and an abundance of fruits and vegetables your top priorities. This strategy aids general health in addition to weight loss.

Encouraging a Sustainable and Balanced Approach to Weight Management

Using a sustainable and balanced strategy is essential for effective weight management. Here are some pointers to help you do this:

i. Make sensible goals: Don't try to lose a lot of weight. Instead, concentrate on long-term, sustainable goals that are reasonable and attainable.

ii. Mindful Eating: Recognize your body's signals of hunger and fullness. Refrain from overindulging in food and exercise portion control.

iii. Consistency Is More vital Than Perfection: Perfection is not as vital as consistency. Periodically indulging is acceptable as long as you get back on track.

To sum up, the secret to success in weight loss is to distinguish truth from myth. Achieving and maintaining a healthy weight requires a well-rounded, evidence-based weight management strategy. We will discuss practical strategies and tips for putting these ideas into practice in your day-to-day activities in the upcoming chapter.

Tracking Progress and Preserving Motivation

As you move forward with your weight loss and management journey, it's imperative to keep track of your progress and stay inspired. This chapter will look at three essential elements of your success: monitoring your progress, setting realistic goals, and maintaining motivation.

Monitoring Your Progress

You must have a clear understanding of your progress if you want to successfully manage your weight. Keeping track of your trip holds you accountable and assists in making the required modifications. This is how you do it:

i. Keep a Journal: To track your daily intake, keep a food journal. You can use this to find trends and places where you can get better. Take note of your workout regimens and your emotional and physical well-being.

ii. Frequent Weigh-Ins: Check your weight frequently, but not compulsively. Usually, a weekly weigh-in will be enough to determine your progress. Remember that there are a lot of reasons why weight can change, so pay attention to patterns over time.

iii. Measurements and Photos: Measure your waist, hips, and other vital places in addition to the scale. Take occasional pictures to visually documented your transformation

Keeping Yourself Motivated

Although motivation can fluctuate, there are ways to maintain it throughout your weight loss journey:

i. Don't forget your "Why": Go back to the reasons you decided to take this trip. Keep your motivations front and center, whether they are greater confidence, better health, or a desire to engage in more physical activity.

ii. Honor accomplishments: Honor your accomplishments before waiting to obtain your ultimate objective. Celebrate and give recognition to the little victories you have along the path.

iii. Remain Responsible: Discuss your objectives with a family member or friend who can encourage you and help you stay responsible. Think about joining a community or group that shares your goals.

To sum up, monitoring your development and maintaining motivation are critical components of your weight reduction and maintenance process. You may continue on the path to success by keeping an eye on your progress, setting reasonable goals, and staying motivated. We'll look at how to deal with obstacles and setbacks and how to get back on track in the upcoming chapter.

Difficulties and Obstacles

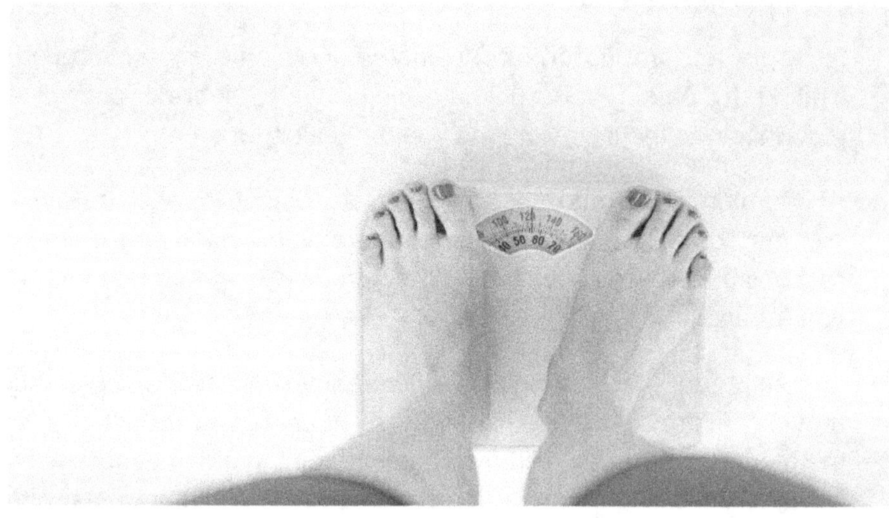

You may probably run across obstacles and reach plateaus in your weight loss and control journey. These situations can be annoying, but you can get through them if you have the correct knowledge and techniques. This chapter will give you ideas for long-term weight management, as well as assist you comprehend weight loss plateaus and how to deal with setbacks.

Recognizing Weight Loss Plateau and Coping Strategies

Obstacles in weight loss are common and can be demoralizing. They appear when, in spite of your continuous efforts, your growth seems to be stagnating. It's important to realize, though, that difficulties are a normal part of the process. This is how you get past them:

i. Evaluate Your Habits: A plateau may be a sign that it's time to reevaluate your activity and nutrition plans. Do you still maintain a calorie deficit, and have you gotten too accustomed to doing out? Make the required modifications.

ii. Vary Your training Schedule: Your body can adjust to training, which will slow down your progress. Try other exercises or up the stakes on your current schedule to provide variation.

iii. Control Stress and Sleep: Stress and insufficient sleep might make it difficult to lose weight. Make rest a priority, concentrate on stress-reduction strategies, and make sure you're getting enough good sleep.

iv. Remain Persistent and Patient: Patience might be tried by plateaus. Keep in mind that they are only temporary, and with time and persistence, you will succeed.

Overcoming Obstacles and Preserving Resilience

An inherent aspect of any weight loss journey is experiencing setbacks. They can manifest in various ways, such as emotional eating or skipping exercise. Here's how to overcome obstacles and maintain your resilience:

i. Acknowledge Reality: Try not to obsess over your errors or failures. Recognize that they are a normal component of learning and that everyone experiences them.

ii. Examine and Learn: Make the most of failures as chances to improve. Examine what went wrong and draw conclusions. Was emotional eating brought on by stress? Did a hectic schedule cause you to miss workouts? Determine the main reasons.

iii. Recommit to Your Goals: Recommit to your goals rather than giving up. Get back your motivation and concentrate on the progress you've achieved so far, which is positive.

Techniques for Maintaining a Healthy Weight Over Time

It's as crucial to maintain your weight reduction progress as it is to reduce your body weight. The following are some long-term weight-maintenance strategies:

i. Livelihood Rather Than Diet: Convert from thinking of your journey as a short-term diet to a long-term way of living. Maintain the healthy routines you've established.

ii. Frequent Check-Ins: Make time to check in with yourself on a regular basis. Make sure your habits and goals are still in line with your present priorities and needs by reevaluating them.

iii. Maintenance Calories: After you reach your goal weight, reduce your calorie consumption to maintenance levels as opposed to a deficit. This stops you from losing more weight.

Iv. Consistent Exercise: To help you maintain your weight and general health, stick to a regular exercise schedule.

In summary, obstacles and plateaus are a natural part of the process of losing and maintaining weight. You can have long-lasting success in your pursuit of a better lifestyle by comprehending and overcoming plateaus, handling setbacks, and putting long-term maintenance techniques into practice. We'll talk about the value of having a supportive community and offer advice on how to locate and create one in the upcoming chapter

Celebrating Success and Maintaining a Healthy Lifestyle

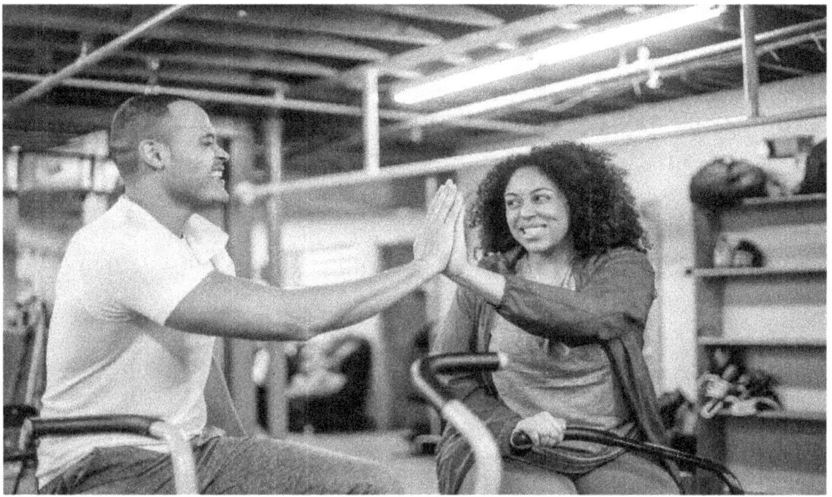

This chapter is all about acknowledging your successes and embracing a sustainable, healthy lifestyle. It's important to celebrate your accomplishments because it will keep you motivated and recognize the hard work you've put into your weight loss and management journey. Here's how to celebrate weight loss milestones:

i. Set Milestone Goals: Divide your weight loss journey into smaller goals, like every 5 or 10 pounds lost. Reward yourself with a non-food treat when you reach a milestone, such as a spa day, a new outfit, or a stress-relieving day at the park.

ii. Share Your Success: Don't be afraid to tell friends and family about your accomplishments; their support and encouragement can be incredibly uplifting and motivating.

iii. Reflect on Your Progress: Take some time to take stock of your progress and realize how far you've come. Keeping a journal or a visual reminder of your accomplishments can help you feel more confident and motivated.

Making the Switch from Losing Weight to Maintaining It

A crucial stage in your journey is moving from active weight loss to weight maintenance.

Here's how to handle this change:

i. Modify Your Energy Consumption: Increase your calorie intake gradually until it reaches maintenance levels. This stabilizes your weight and stops you from losing any more.

ii. Maintain Healthy Habits: You should keep up the routines you established during your weight loss period, such as consistent exercise and a well-balanced diet.

iii. Observe and Modify: Pay attention to your weight. To keep your weight where you want it, modify as needed if you see changes.

Ultimately, acknowledging and appreciating your accomplishments, shifting from weight reduction to maintenance, and making a lifetime commitment to health and wellness represent the latter stages of your journey. You may live a longer, healthier, and more satisfying life by acknowledging and appreciating your accomplishments, leading a sustainable, balanced lifestyle, and making a commitment to your well-being. Congrats on your weight reduction and weight control journey.

Conclusion: Starting Your Path to Health and Well-Being

We've looked at the difficult but worthwhile journey of weight loss and management in this eBook. We've dispelled myths, addressed important issues, and offered advice based on the best available research to assist you in reaching and maintaining a healthy weight along the way. It's time to compile and highlight the most important lessons learned so you may take charge of your own weight control journey.

Highlighting the Main Ideas from the Book

You've learned insightful tips and useful tactics for effective weight management throughout the book:

i. Knowing Your Why: Never forget the motivations behind your decision to take this trip. Your inspiration will serve as your guide.

ii. Balanced Nutrition: Give top priority to a diet rich in fruits, vegetables, whole grains, lean meats, and healthy fats. Portion control and mindful eating are essential.

iii. Regular Exercise: To improve your general health and control your weight, mix strength and cardio activities into your program.

iv. Tracking Progress: To stay on course and make necessary corrections, log your journey using measurements, a journal, and frequent weigh-ins.

v. Celebrating Success: Honor your accomplishments, no matter how modest they may appear. Treat yourself to something sweet to help you stay motivated.

We encourage you to start your own weight control journey with increased information and confidence as you close this eBook. Recall that it has nothing to do with drastic diets or fast remedies. It's about making lifelong, healthful decisions that will benefit you.

Despite the fact that every trip is different and every road has its share of obstacles, you are now more equipped than ever with the skills and information you've learned from this book. You possess the ability to design a life that is healthier, happier, and more satisfying for yourself.

You have the resources to be successful whether your objective is weight loss, maintenance, or just adopting a better lifestyle.

Reaches and obstacles should not discourage you; rather, they should be viewed as chances for development and education. Your path to a better, happier self is a lifetime marathon, not a sprint.

An addition

We've provided a guide with more resources, including suggested reading lists, schedules for exercise, and sample meal plans, to help you on your journey. These resources are intended to give you useful tools to support you on your journey to wellbeing and weight control.

We appreciate you using this eBook as a roadmap to help you become a better, happier version of yourself. We hope your quest for a more happy and health-conscious existence is successful. May prosperity, joy, and the bliss of wellbeing envelop your path.